THE LITTLE
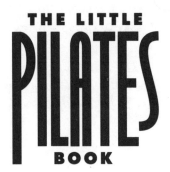
PILATES
BOOK

THE LITTLE
PILATES
BOOK

ERIKA DILLMAN

WARNER BOOKS

A Time Warner Company

Neither these pilates exercises and programs nor any other exercise program should be followed without first consulting a health care professional. If you have any special conditions requiring attention, you should consult with your health care professional regularly regarding possible modifications of the program contained in this book.

Copyright © 2001 by Erika Dillman
All rights reserved.

Warner Books, Inc., 1271 Avenue of the Americas, New York, NY 10020

Visit our Web site at www.twbookmark.com.

For information on Time Warner Trade Publishing's online publishing program, visit www.ipublish.com.

 A Time Warner Company

Printed in the United States of America

First Printing: July 2001

10 9 8 7 6 5 4 3 2 1

Library of Congress Cataloging-in-Publication Data

Dillman, Erika
  The little pilates book / Erika Dillman.
    p. cm.
  Includes index.
  ISBN 0-446-67827-9
  1. Pilates method. 2. Exercise. 3. Physical fitness. I. Title.

RA781.D53 2001
613.7'1—dc21   2001017942

Book design and text composition by L&G McRee
Text illustrations by Jim Chow

For Maddie and Jack

Acknowledgments

I would like to thank the following people for their contributions to *The Little Pilates Book:*

My agent Anne Depue, my editor Diana Baroni, and assistant editor Molly Chehak for believing in my books.

The Pilates instructors who generously shared their time and expertise with me: Jane Erskine, Lauren Stephen, Stephanie Cusik, and Patricia Kaminski.

My friends Eileen McKeough, Kathy Mack, and Terence Pagard for their editorial suggestions and for test-driving all of the exercises.

Joan Breibart, president of the PhysicalMind Institute, for providing research information.

Jim Chow for his wonderful illustrations.

My friends and family for their encouragement and support.

Contents

Welcome to
The Little Pilates Book

If you're interested in health and fitness, you've probably heard about the "new" exercise called Pilates, and you might be wondering if it's the right exercise for you.

Certainly, the benefits of practicing Pilates exercises sound almost too good to be true: achieving a flatter, stronger stomach; better posture; a reduction in lower back pain; and developing a strong, toned body without getting bulky muscles.

So how do you get started? Who can practice Pilates? Is it difficult to learn? Can you practice Pilates at home?

My goals are to answer these common questions and explain the key concepts of the Pilates exercise method, with a minimum of jargon and no hype. This book is for anyone, regardless of age, gender, or experience, who wants to improve her or his fitness level and enjoy better health. In addition to learning how to perform the Pilates exercises, I hope you gain a better understanding of how your body functions during movement so that you can begin to lay the groundwork for a lifetime of fitness.

In *The Little Pilates Book,* you'll learn about the different applications of Pilates exercises, how to get started with your own mat routine, the benefits you can gain by practicing regularly at home, how to get "fab abs," and some of the fundamentals of posture and alignment. I've also included definitions of common Pilates terms, as well as instructions for a complete Pilates mat workout, including tips to help you better understand the movements and positions for each exercise.

As with any new undertaking, there is a learning curve involved with becoming proficient at Pilates. Remember to take your time, be patient and kind to yourself, and above all, have fun. I hope this book will help make your transition smoother. With persistence and practice, you, too, will be able to move through life with strength and grace.

—ERIKA DILLMAN

1 | My Pilates Journey

When I first started hearing about Pilates, I was skeptical. I figured it was just another trendy exercise program that promised results but didn't deliver. I also had no idea how to pronounce Pilates until I saw a phonetic spelling (puh-la-tees) in a magazine article.

The fact that dancers and movie stars swore by Pilates just made me more suspicious. I'd seen too many infomercials in which Hollywood celebrities hawked every type of "miracle" gadget meant to tone abs, butts, and thighs . . . "in just three minutes a day!" And who can trust dancers, anyway? They can do things with their bodies that we normal people could never imagine. Pilates was just a passing fad. It wasn't for me. Or so I thought.

THE EXERCISE FOR ME

No, Pilates wasn't for me . . . until my health club opened a Pilates studio, and my curiosity got the best of me. Every time I walked past the studio, I tried to see what was going on in there, but room dividers blocked the windows so that peepers like me didn't disturb the people inside.

Then I heard women talking about Pilates in the locker room. I got jealous. Were they using the new studio? Was it fun in there? What did they have that I didn't have? Why did they get to use the new equipment and I didn't? Were they in better shape than me? Suddenly, my exercise routine seemed stale and ineffective; I wanted in that room. I needed to be in that room. And yet, a part of me still doubted that this was the exercise for me. I'm not a stretchy person or a strong person, and I don't like to exercise in groups.

FIRST CLASS

I decided to start with a group mat class. When I arrived, I had no idea what to expect. I gave the other people in the class—

four women and one man—a good looking over, and decided that I was younger and fitter than most of them. It couldn't be that hard.

In the next hour, a small, incredibly strong and flexible woman led us through a series of challenging exercises. Of course, I was humbled when everyone in the class looked better doing the exercises than I did. I had a little trouble keeping up and knowing whether or not I was doing the exercises correctly. Thankfully, my yoga background came in handy. Many of the exercises seemed very similar to yoga poses.

I liked that all of the exercises we practiced were done while lying on our backs, stomachs, or sides on a thick mat. Not having to stand up was great for me. I had a variety of health problems, including sinus problems and low blood pressure, which often made exercising while standing up very difficult.

My favorite thing about Pilates was that all of the exercises focused on my abs, my middle. I'd been complaining for a few years about my bulging gut and love handles, yet I hadn't found exercises that I could do to address those problems. My usual exercise, running, was temporarily on the back burner due to a foot injury. And crunches had never worked for me; I always felt uncomfortable doing them.

By the time the class ended, I was pretty tired, but I had made it through the workout without humiliating or harming myself! I felt like the space between my pelvis and rib cage had lengthened, and I could see how, with practice, I could strengthen my torso and improve my posture. The next day it was obvious that my body had received a big wake-up call; muscles I didn't even know I had were sore.

ONE ON ONE

I decided to take some private lessons in addition to attending group mat classes so that I could gain a better understanding of the routine, as well as improve my form.

Working one-on-one with an instructor made all the difference. She explained how to correctly perform the exercises, making modifications where I needed them. Despite my flabby abs, I was a quick study.

Pilates made me keenly aware of my body's imbalances. I was overusing some muscles and underusing others. Like most people, I'd always neglected working my core muscles. My instructor helped me understand the link between having a strong core and good posture.

With time and practice, the post-exercise soreness I experienced after my first few classes went away. I still felt a bit sore the day after a Pilates workout. My muscles weren't painful, but they were making their presence known. The exercises continued to challenge me, but I always left every session walking a bit taller.

I decided that Pilates *was* for me.

2 | What Is Pilates?

THE METHOD

Pilates is an exercise method designed to condition and connect body and mind, correct muscle imbalances, improve posture, and tone the body.

Created by German fitness trainer Joseph H. Pilates more than seventy years ago, Pilates is based on a combination of eastern and western exercise philosophies. The exercises mix yoga-like movements with strengthening techniques to develop strong, lean, flexible muscles.

Pilates exercises, which are sometimes referred to as "the

method," are organized and practiced sequentially. Each exercise is linked to and builds upon the previous exercise to achieve total body strength and greater mind-body awareness. Movements are practiced with control and precision, with an emphasis on achieving correct form, rather than performing endless repetitions.

There are many applications of Pilates; it can be done on a mat and/or using specially designed machines and apparatuses. Including the different applications and many modifications, there are nearly five hundred Pilates exercises, although only twenty to thirty are relevant to the beginning and intermediate level students for whom this book is written.

The Little Pilates Book focuses on Pilates mat work, the most accessible form of the exercise system since it requires no equipment and can be practiced anywhere.

THE CORE

The primary focus of Pilates is to strengthen the body's core, the area between your hips and sternum. Pilates instructors often refer to this area as your "powerhouse" because, as you may already know, your body's center is the source of your power, balance, and movement.

The core muscles include spinal muscles, inner thigh muscles, psoas muscles (muscles that run from the spine through the pelvis and attach to the inner thighs, linking the upper and lower body), and four layers of abdominal muscles. These muscles work together to support the spine, which, in turn, promotes good posture. Pilates works the deepest layers of these muscles, as well as the hamstrings, quadriceps, and glutes (butt muscles). (See page 11 for a body map that shows the locations of some basic muscle groups.)

When your core isn't strong, you lack the torso stability to fully access your power and move efficiently. You may be relying more on your arm, leg, or back muscles to provide support or balance when you try to move. That means that your limbs are not able to move efficiently and your back may be strained. After time, you'll develop muscle imbalances, poor postural habits, and even lower back pain.

Practicing Pilates exercises helps strengthen core muscles uniformly so that they provide the support and balance your spine needs to maintain good posture. With good posture, your limbs are free to move as they were intended. The ultimate goal

BASIC MUSCLE GROUPS
Figure 2.1

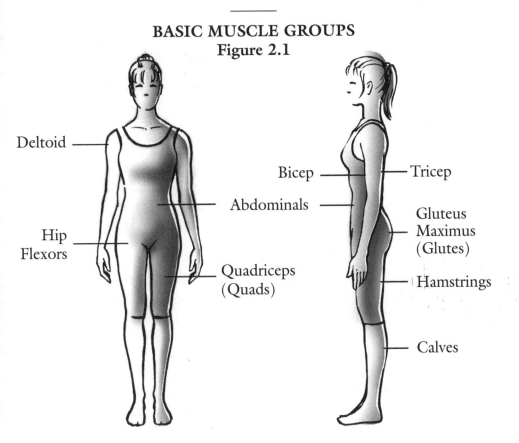

Deltoid

Bicep — Tricep

Abdominals

Gluteus
Maximus
(Glutes)

Hip
Flexors

Quadriceps
(Quads)

Hamstrings

Calves

of Pilates exercises is to integrate core strength with flexible limbs (and joints) for a balanced, full-body workout.

BENEFITS OF PRACTICE

There's a reason Pilates has become so popular in the past few years—it works. Pilates is an efficient, effective exercise method that actually addresses the areas of the body that most of us would like to tone up: the stomach, thighs, and butt. You don't need any special equipment to do the mat exercises, and you don't have to join a gym.

Many people are tired of going to the gym, jumping around, and spending time on exercises that don't produce results. Pilates offers people an exercise routine that is focused, self-directed, and helps them get more in touch with their bodies.

The main purpose of Pilates is to restore optimal functioning to the body. It can be used as a conditioning exercise and/or as part of a rehabilitative physical therapy program. Practiced regularly, and with correct form, Pilates can help you achieve many physical and emotional benefits, including:

What Is Pilates?

- Stronger abdominal muscles
- Improved posture
- Reduced risk of lower back pain and other injuries
- Increased total body strength without developing bulky muscles
- Increased flexibility and joint mobility
- Improved endurance
- Improved concentration, coordination, and balance
- Increased mind-body awareness
- Greater confidence
- Increased energy
- Aid in injury recovery

When your body is strong and balanced, no longer limited by muscle weaknesses and imbalances, you'll walk taller and move with more efficiency and grace. You'll also look and feel more confident and more comfortable, and your stomach, thighs, and butt will look toned and trim.

If you're active in recreational activities and sports, the improved balance, strength, and centeredness you can gain from Pilates will help you prevent injuries and improve your performance. If you're new to exercise, you'll gain a better understanding of how your body functions, as well as a sense of control over your body that you might have been lacking. Improving your posture and fitness level will also improve your circulation and breathing, reenergizing your body and mind.

WHO PRACTICES PILATES?

Anyone who wants to improve her or his fitness level, appearance, and overall health can practice Pilates. It's the perfect exercise for women, men, seniors, teens, athletes, and people new to exercise or recovering from injuries.

Since Pilates was first taught and practiced in the United States in the early 1920s, movie stars, dancers, and athletes have sworn by it. Everyone from Gregory Peck and Katharine Hepburn, to Julia Roberts and Glenn Close, to Australian tennis pro Pat Cash, have used Pilates as part of their fitness regimens.

Dancers especially have been drawn to the Pilates method because it allows them to increase their flexibility and strength without creating bulky muscles. Athletes often use Pilates to help correct muscle imbalances and increase their abdominal strength and overall power. For actors, whose appearance can be crucial to career success, Pilates offers an effective workout that can give them long, toned muscles, a flatter stomach, and enhance their physical agility and poise.

Pilates is ideal for anyone with a busy schedule because it can be done anywhere, and at twenty to forty-five minutes a workout, it fits easily into your day. People who sit or stand all day and/or who use a computer can also benefit from Pilates because the exercises help counteract the physical and emotional stresses your body endures every day.

PILATES MAT WORK

Pilates mat exercises are considered by many Pilates experts to be the core of the method. A typical Pilates workout might include ten to twenty exercises that are performed on a thick mat or on the floor.

All of the exercises are done while lying on your back, stomach, or side, or from a sitting position so that there is no impact or stress on the joints. Many of the movements may look familiar to you if you've done yoga or other mat-based exercises.

Pilates is based on the theory that a few correctly executed movements produce benefits. Therefore, when practicing, you only repeat each exercise a few times before moving on to the next exercise. The challenge in practicing Pilates mat work is to concentrate on every movement so that you perform the exercises fluidly using control and precision.

You can practice mat work at home (it's recommended that you take a few lessons from a certified instructor first to learn correct form). If you need more instruction, attend private or group mat-work classes at a Pilates studio or at a health club that offers Pilates instruction.

Once you learn the correct form, you can train yourself, exercising wherever you have enough space to lie down. For many people group mat classes are a much more affordable option than private lessons in mat work or in using the machines. The different types of Pilates instruction available will be discussed further in Chapter 7.

PILATES, YOGA, AND AEROBIC EXERCISE

Pilates is most often compared to both yoga and strength training. Understanding the similarities and differences between Pilates and these other two exercise methods can help you clarify what you want to gain from Pilates.

Like yoga, Pilates is concerned with connecting mind and body; improving muscle strength, tone, and flexibility; developing good posture; and improving breathing. Most people turn to yoga for its physical benefits, but there is a spiritual element to the practice that some yoga students pursue. In its purest form, the goal of yoga exercises is to prepare the body for meditation, although most classes in the United States focus mainly on the physical aspects of yoga.

Pilates, on the other hand, requires mindfulness during practice, but the exercises are an end in themselves. Performing them with control, precision, and flowing movements is the ultimate goal. Pilates is not concerned with spiritual matters, although you may feel your spirits lift as you become stronger and more fit.

Strength training (i.e., weight lifting) is another exercise incorporated in the Pilates method. Weight lifting, usually performed with weight machines, builds lean muscle mass, burns fat, and increases bone density. Pilates also develops lean muscles and promotes healthy bones, but uses your own body weight for resistance.

Unlike weight lifting, Pilates exercises allow the limbs to move through their full range of motion, which stretches and lengthens muscles as well as improving joint mobility for a more integrated type of strength that directly relates to movement.

In Pilates, you isolate different body parts during an exercise, while stabilizing the body with your core muscles. The positions in Pilates exercises were designed this way so that the movements of the limbs become coordinated with the center of the body, promoting more efficient and powerful movements.

Pilates is a well-rounded exercise in itself and complements aerobic exercises such as walking, running, biking, and swimming, as well as sports. Following a Pilates routine with a short yoga routine is a great way to take advantage of your core strength and create greater muscle length and flexibility. As you progress to intermediate and advanced level Pilates workouts, you'll see that Pilates can also be an aerobic exercise. If you're trying to lose weight, remember that both diet and exercise play a role. Weight loss occurs when you burn more calories than you consume.

No More Crunches

I can't think of anyone who likes doing crunches, but everyone I know would like a flatter stomach. With Pilates you can condition your abdominal muscles without doing dozens of repetitions or straining your neck.

Pilates exercises like The Roll-Up (page 96) are actually more effective and safer than crunches. Here are a few of the major differences between The Roll-Up and the crunch:

- *Range of Motion*
Roll-Ups move the spine through a full forward flexion (bending). Crunches require only partial forward flexion. Full forward flexion helps improve the range of motion in the spine and develops abdominal muscles more effectively.

- *Long Muscles*
The Roll-Up works the abdominal muscles at different

lengths as the spine moves through its full range of motion. The result is muscles with more length, control, flexibility, and endurance, helping create space between the pelvis and rib cage for a long, lean look.

• *Positioning*

In The Roll-Up, the abdominal muscles are used to move through the exercise, and the position of the body allows the legs to remain relaxed. When doing crunches, it's easy to rely on leg or hip muscles, or to pull on the head with the hands, to execute the movement.

• *Pace*

The Roll-Up is performed more slowly than crunches, relying on control and precision to move the trunk through its full forward flexion (and back down to the floor again). Crunches are usually performed quickly, making it easy to relax the abs as the body is lowered toward the floor (but not to the floor) and to rely on momentum to raise the body rather than abdominal strength or control.

(Source: PhysicalMind Institute)

3 | Philosophy and Origins of Pilates

"Physical fitness is the first requisite to happiness."
—JOSEPH H. PILATES

JOSEPH H. PILATES (1880–1967)

It's hard to think of an exercise enthusiast as fervent in his beliefs as Joseph Hubertus Pilates, a German fitness trainer who, in the early 1900s, created "Contrology," the exercise method we now call Pilates.

After a childhood plagued by illness and frailty, the young Pilates, determined to be strong and active, devoted himself to building up his weak body. He became proficient in a variety of sports, including strength training, diving, gymnastics, skiing, and boxing.

During this period of physical transformation Pilates began to form his philosophies about exercise and health. From his study of yoga, acrobatics, and animal movements—to name just a few of his influences—he developed his theories on movement and fitness, blending philosophies of eastern and western health practices and exercises.

Pilates used to say that his ideas were fifty years ahead of his time, and indeed, this message still rings true today. Pick up any health and fitness magazine and you'll read the same advice that Pilates extolled in the early 1920s—to live a happy life, you need to take care of your body and mind through exercise and healthy living.

RETURN TO LIFE

In his 1945 book, *Return to Life*, Pilates outlined in zealous detail the purpose and goals of his exercise method. He believed that the stresses of modern life (e.g., working in offices, living in cities, breathing polluted air, lacking social or relaxation time) were detrimental to physical fitness and well-being.

For Pilates, the pursuit of health and fitness was not only a physical and emotional responsibility, but a moral responsibility as well. He lived by, and often quoted, the Roman motto, "mens sana in corpore sano," which means "a sound mind in a sound body." By practicing his exercise method, people could "return to life," regaining harmony and balance in the body, as well as peace and calm in the mind.

Contrology, or Pilates, as it is now called, was a holistic exercise plan that required people to take responsibility for their well-being by adhering to a disciplined, focused system of exercises. Pilates' plan included performing these exercises faithfully on a regular basis, using concentration, control, and precision to execute the various movements.

Pilates exercises were designed not only to strengthen, stretch, and tone the body, but to improve breathing, concentration, and coordination in the body. The goals of the method included increasing circulation, correcting muscle and postural imbalances, and restoring vitality to body and mind. The ultimate goal was a body that could endure the stresses of modern life and still have energy left to enjoy recreation and time with friends and family.

Exercise was, of course, central to the plan, but Pilates also encouraged people to adopt healthier habits like getting enough sleep every night, setting aside time for relaxation and visiting friends, and eating a healthy diet. Pilates noticed that as many people aged they continued to eat the same hearty meals that they had eaten when they lived a much more active life. He believed that a person should eat only enough food to fuel his body for its daily activities.

DEVELOPING THE METHOD

Pilates studied obsessively, constantly honing his ideas and methods to develop what he considered the perfect exercise for body and mind. He got a chance to test his methods and theories during World War I.

In the years before the war Pilates lived in England, working as a self-defense trainer, boxer, and circus performer. When the war broke out, Pilates was interned with other German nationals. In the camp he trained the other internees in his mat work. Some people in the health and fitness world have speculated that Pilates' exercise regimen may have helped the internees stay strong and healthy, protecting them from the influenza epidemic of 1918. While thousands died in London, not one internee succumbed to the disease.

After the war, Pilates returned to Germany and worked as a hospital orderly. During this period, he continued to develop his exercise method. Using bed springs, he rigged up hospital beds to create exercise machines. These bed contraptions allowed patients with injuries and illnesses to exercise without getting out of bed or further injuring themselves.

Pilates didn't stay in Germany long. After rejecting a job as the fitness trainer for the German army, Pilates headed for the United States. When he landed in New York he opened up an exercise studio with his wife, Clara, who shared his passion for health and exercise.

It didn't take long for the word to get out about Pilates' exercise method. Dancers flocked to his New York studio. The exercises were perfectly suited to dancers because they could develop strength without adding bulk. The Pilates method was also an ideal rehabilitative exercise since it allowed injured dancers to exercise without straining existing injuries. Among his loyal followers were some of the world's most famous dancers and performing artists, including Martha Graham, George Balanchine, and Hanya Holm.

Today Pilates' theories remain the foundation of modern Pilates teacher training and instruction.

4 | Guiding Principles

In order to create real change in your body and improve your fitness level, it's important to understand not only the movements involved in Pilates exercises but the guiding principles that take this simple mat exercise and transform it into a holistic, restorative, mind-body workout.

Following these eight basic guidelines will help you understand the form and intent of the different exercises so that you can begin to learn more about your body and how it functions during movement. With this new understanding and regular practice, you'll soon internalize these exercise principles, helping you establish healthy movement patterns and preparing you for a lifetime of fitness.

1) CONCENTRATION

*"Concentrate on the correct movements EACH TIME YOU EX-
ERCISE, lest you do them improperly and thus lose all the vital
benefits of their value."*

—JOSEPH H. PILATES

It's easy when you lift weights, run on a treadmill, or go to an
aerobics class to tune out and just go through the motions. Unfortunately, distracting yourself with music or mirroring your
fitness instructor's moves separates your mind from your
movements. And that usually means that you're not paying attention to your form. In Pilates, form is everything, and in
order to practice your exercises in correct form, you need to put
your mind to the task.

Developing a greater awareness about how your body moves,
which muscle groups initiate specific movement, and how to
coordinate your movements with your breath will help you address muscle imbalances, weakness, and other postural problems. Concentrating while performing the exercises will help
retrain your body and mind to restore healthy movement patterns that promote optimal functioning.

Visualization is another way that your mind helps train your body. You'll notice in the exercise instructions in Chapter 8 that many include descriptions of visual images to help you understand specific movements. When you're learning a new exercise, it can be difficult to locate and use your muscles in a new way. Visualizing helps the brain and nervous system recruit the right muscles for the job.

2) CONTROL

"Contrology begins with mind control over muscles."
—JOSEPH H. PILATES

Controlled movement is another key element of the Pilates method. Maintaining control throughout your workout is essential to performing the exercises in correct form. In turn, it is through correct form that you prevent injuries and build strong, lean, functional muscles.

If you didn't exercise with control, your body would go into default mode, using momentum to perform the exercises or relying on your strongest muscles (i.e., old, unhealthy patterns) to move through each exercise. Using control, you exercise both major and minor muscle groups, strengthening, lengthening, and toning the body in a more effective, balanced way.

As you practice Pilates, you need to concentrate on your position, and on the movement you intend to make. You'll notice that the mat exercises are done on the floor, holding the torso still while moving the arms and legs. First you stabilize the torso and lower back by engaging your abdominal muscles, then, you make controlled movements with your arms and legs and sometimes with the upper body. If you can focus your mind and control your movement to stay in correct form, you'll be on your way to reaping the benefits of Pilates.

3) Precision and Coordination

"Correctly executed and mastered to the point of subconscious reaction, these exercises will reflect grace and balance in your routine activities."

—Joseph H. Pilates

Think of an ice skater, twirling on one foot, then jumping high into the air, then spinning in circles. What makes watching her so fascinating is the precision and gracefulness with which she moves. Although she makes it look effortless, we know that behind that grace is years of training, and incredible power and strength.

Like skating, Pilates is about making the right movements with the right muscles at the right pace. The entire body is interconnected, and each movement is the result of a series of messages that originate in the brain, travel along the nerves, and finally, tell the muscles how and when to move. Concentrating on this process so that you can practice your exercises in correct form is one more aspect of developing mind-body awareness.

Most people feel uncoordinated when they try a new sport or exercise, and that's normal because their bodies have no memory of the movements they are trying to make. Focusing on the correct form will help train your body and mind, increasing your coordination, balance, and muscle tone.

Practicing exercises that demand coordination is as good for the brain as it is for the muscles, ligaments, and joints. The Swimming exercise (page 144) is a perfect example of how precision and coordination are used in Pilates. As you lie on your stomach, stabilizing your lower back with your abdominal muscles, you raise your right arm and left leg at the same time, then switch positions, raising your left arm and right leg. This type of cross-lateral training requires both sides of the brain to work together.

Quality of movement, not quantity, is important in Pilates. As you work to integrate muscles and mind, continue to focus on control and coordination.

4) ISOLATION AND INTEGRATION

"Each muscle may cooperatively and loyally aid in the uniform development of all of our muscles."

—JOSEPH H. PILATES

Increasing flexibility without sacrificing strength is one of the primary benefits of Pilates. One way to increase flexibility is to develop the weaker, underutilized muscles in muscle pairs. If you look at the Side Kick on page 137, you'll see that you first extend your leg forward, then you bring your leg behind the body. Each movement places emphasis on different muscles and also requires several muscles to work together. By exercising weaker muscles as well as the stronger muscles, you'll create more balance in your body, which will help you make controlled, precise movements.

In order to develop weaker muscles, you need to isolate the joints. For example, when you do the Single Leg Circle (page 100), several things must happen at once in order for you to succeed and gain benefits from the exercise. Your core needs to be stable, with your torso planted on the floor, while your leg moves through its motion with control and precision. Using your abdominal muscles to stabilize your lower back, you isolate your hip so that you primarily use your hip and leg muscles to rotate your leg.

If you don't maintain abdominal control, your body will unintentionally recruit the wrong muscles to move your leg, which could result in injury.

Pilates exercises help integrate muscles to work together, not only in muscle pairs, but throughout the entire body. As you integrate your core with the more superficial big movement muscles of the limbs, you use less energy to move your limbs, allowing for stronger, more flexible joints. This type of conditioning relates directly to the many different movements you'll make in all of your daily activities. With Pilates, you train your core muscles to support your body in its upright position and balance so that your arms and legs can function more efficiently.

5) CENTERING

"Good posture can be successfully acquired only when the entire mechanism of the body is under perfect control."
—JOSEPH H. PILATES

In Pilates, you work from the inside out, developing the core, or abdominal, muscles so that they can function as intended—to support the spine and the internal organs, as well as move the torso.

If you are familiar with other exercises like yoga, t'ai chi, or karate, you might already know that all movement originates from your core. Literally and figuratively, it is your body's source of power, balance, and strength.

The goal of Pilates is to develop abdominal strength, endurance, and control in order to maintain good posture and prepare the body to perform all of its daily activities. Core strength is essential for every movement you make, whether it's working on a computer, playing tennis, or schussing down a ski slope.

If you spend most of your days sitting at a desk and you have weak, unconditioned abdominal muscles, you'll develop poor postural habits that eventually could cause pain and injury in your neck, back, or other parts of your body. If you try to play your favorite sports with weak abs, you won't be as powerful or effective in your game.

Think of the movements involved in swinging a baseball bat. If you stand in one place and only move your arms, swatting at the ball, you won't hit the ball very hard or very far and you'll have a hard time hitting the ball in the direction you want it to go. But if you integrate and coordinate your movements, stepping into your swing, and rotating the torso as you bring your arms through a full swing, you'll be able to crack a line drive down the third base line. It's as if there's a ball of energy in your center, and when you move, it sends energy forward and out to the limbs.

You'll notice in Chapter 8 that all of the Pilates exercises include instructions to "pull your abs to your spine," a move that stabilizes your spine and lower back in preparation for moving your limbs or torso. When you make this movement, you want to locate the rectus abdominis, the abdominal muscle that runs vertically from your pubic bone to your sternum, and pull it in toward the spine. Imagine that you are laying the muscles against the spine, beginning at the pubic bone until you reach the sternum. Think strength and length.

At the same time, you want to feel your other abdominal muscles, which form a kind of corset around your waist, wrapping around your waist toward your back. Using the abdominal muscles in this way helps build strength, endurance, and control, allowing you to lengthen and stretch your spine while protecting the lower back.

You'll read more about the abdominal muscles in Chapter 5.

6) FLOWING MOVEMENT

"Contrology is designed to give you suppleness, natural grace, and skill that will be unmistakably reflected in the way you walk, in the way you play, and in the way you work."
—JOSEPH H. PILATES

Pilates exercises are meant to be performed in one flowing movement. Initially, you'll spend time on each exercise just trying to coordinate all of the different movements and positions. With practice, you'll soon develop a rhythm that carries you from one exercise to the next. This doesn't mean that you'll mindlessly sail through your workout; you still have to concentrate on every move.

As you practice your exercises, try not to make any sudden, jerky movements, but stay relaxed and focused, lengthening through the torso and limbs with every extension. Think of Pilates as a dance—with each movement leading gracefully into the next.

7) BREATHING

"To breathe correctly you must completely exhale and inhale, always trying very hard to 'squeeze' every atom of impure air from your lungs in much the same manner that you would wring every drop of water from a wet cloth."
—JOSEPH H. PILATES

Breathing is an important element of Pilates. Many of us don't breathe correctly, and we don't even know it. We breathe out of the tops of our lungs, or worse, hold our breath when we move. No wonder we're so tired.

Breathing correctly, fully inhaling and exhaling for a complete exchange of fresh air for stale air, helps maintain blood circulation, supplying the body with oxygen, and carrying away waste products. Pilates will help you get back in touch with the fact that breathing involves your lungs, your diaphragm, and your rib cage. With practice, you'll develop the muscles that help you fully expand your rib cage and chest.

It's easy to forget to breathe when you first begin Pilates. You're so busy trying to remember which muscles to engage and which muscles to relax that you just hold your breath. With time, you'll be able to coordinate your breath with your movements. You'll notice that breathing helps you stay relaxed so that you can safely stretch and move.

As a general rule, you will inhale before initiating movement, or when extending the body, and you will exhale as you initiate movement or bend forward. Exhaling as you move forward or twist the torso helps you relax into the stretch.

8) ROUTINE

"Through repetition you acquire natural rhythm."
—JOSEPH H. PILATES

As with any exercise or sport, you need to practice Pilates regularly to gain benefits.

It takes days, weeks, months, or even years of repetitive negative stresses on the body (such as poor postural habits, injuries, deconditioning, stress) to create the muscle imbalances that cause aches, pains, and injuries. As you read earlier in this chapter, for movement to occur, the brain sends a message to the nerves, which then tell the muscles to move. This nerve circuit between brain and muscles is called a neuromuscular pathway.

Over time, if you develop muscle imbalances that create misalignment in the body, new pathways become established to support those muscles even though they're contributing to poor posture and movement patterns. Then, every time you move, the nerves recruit the same muscles, which keeps you stuck in less than optimal movement patterns.

Pilates exercises are designed to realign the body and uniformly condition muscles so that the right muscles are used in the way they were meant to be used to support and move the body. Repeating movements in correct form helps reestablish new pathways that help the brain and nerves recruit the right muscles for specific movements.

In other words, the more you practice, incorporating all eight of the guidelines, the more you'll be training your brain, nerves, and muscles to establish new movement patterns that promote posture, alignment, and strength.

5 | Posture, Alignment, and Movement

STAND UP STRAIGHT

We all know good posture when we see it (usually in other people), but what does it really mean to "stand up straight" and why is good posture so important?

I've spent most of my life walking around looking like a little question mark—with a swayed lower back and hunched upper back. Unfortunately, my mother's admonitions to "stand up straight" when I was a child fell on deaf ears. I had developed the perfect slouchy posture to express my preadolescent disdain and ennui, and I wasn't about to straighten up for the sake of appearance. I wish now, after a number of back and neck problems, that I had.

It's true that people with good posture look confident and poised, but good posture is so much more than appearance. It's about helping your body function optimally.

Posture and Alignment

Good posture is the vertical alignment of the body. It's important because correct alignment allows your body to move efficiently. In order to achieve vertical alignment of the body, muscles, ligaments, bones, and joints must all function together to maintain balance, perform movements, and hold the body upright.

Looking at the front view of the body (see posture examples on page 43), you can see that an imaginary vertical line runs like an axis through the body from the top of the head, through the center of the body, to the floor, with the nose, chin, sternum, navel, and pubic bone all in one line. The horizonal lines on the figure also help you see that the shoulders are relaxed and in their natural position, indicated by a line parallel to

Figure 5.1

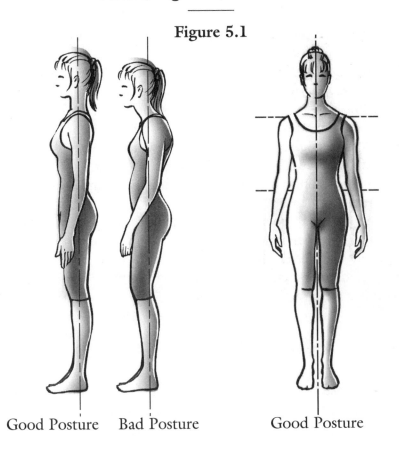

Good Posture   Bad Posture   Good Posture

the floor and to the line across the hips, which shows the pelvis in its natural position.

It's the same with a side view of the body. Notice how the ear, shoulder, elbow, hip, knee, and ankle all fall on the same vertical line. These external landmarks indicate that internally the body is in alignment. The head is sitting on top of the neck, eyes looking straight forward; the spine, with its natural curves, is long and aligned; the pelvis is in its correct position; the limbs are straight but not locked at the joints; and the feet firmly planted on the ground.

When you are in correct alignment, your body is more flexible, your movements more efficient, and your balance and coordination are better. You should be able to maintain good posture and alignment whether you are sitting, standing, or performing other activities or sports.

EFFECTS OF POOR POSTURE

It's no surprise that 80 percent of people will experience some type of back pain in their lives. Most of us have at least a few bad postural habits that contribute to compacting the spine and

**LOOK IN THE MIRROR TO ASSESS YOUR POSTURE.
CAN YOU ANSWER "YES" TO THESE POSTURE GUIDELINES?**

- Is there space between your shoulders and ears?
- Is your head held straight?
- Are your shoulders and hips parallel with each other and with the floor?
- Is the space between your arms and torso equal on both sides?
- Are your kneecaps facing forward?
- Are your ankles parallel to the floor?

Have a friend take a picture of you from a side view, and study your alignment again:

- Is your head held high? Is your ear in line with your shoulder? Is your chin parallel to the floor, or does it tilt too far forward or backward?
- Are your shoulders in line with your ears, or are they pulled back too far or hunched forward?
- Is your chest slightly raised? Is your upper back straight, or hunched over?
- Is your stomach flat? Are your abdominal muscles slightly engaged?
- Does your lower back have a slight natural curve, or is it too flat or too curved forward?
- Are your legs straight without locking your knees?

(Source: American Physical Therapy Association)

creating muscle imbalances. When you add injuries, illnesses, working at a computer, sitting all day, and simply the effects of gravity, there are many factors that can interfere with good posture.

Because the body is interconnected, when one part of the body is out of alignment, it affects the entire structure. When you have poor posture, your bones are not aligned correctly, and that strains your muscles, ligaments, and joints. Poor posture can also impact the internal organs, affecting how they function and even how you breathe. Imbalances and misalignment can cause fatigue and, eventually, pain in your neck, back, hips, or other parts of your body. Poor posture also puts you at greater risk of injury when participating in sports or other recreational activities.

How Pilates Can Help

When the body is not in alignment, minor muscles try to do the work of major muscles, or the same few muscles try to compensate and do all the work of maintaining posture and moving. Pilates helps restore good posture by correcting muscle imbalances, improving joint mobility, increasing flexibility, and strengthening postural muscles.

- Muscles work in pairs, and Pilates is designed to develop your muscles equally so that you build strength in a balanced way. You'll train both major and minor muscle groups so that all of the body's muscles can work together to function the way they were intended. Strong muscles help hold the body upright.

- Flexible muscles are also important in maintaining good posture and supporting the back when still or moving. Without flexibility, movement is limited. Pilates exercises stretch the muscles of the back, abdomen, hips, and limbs.

- Your joints need to be flexible and strong so that you can move and maintain alignment at the same time. Practicing Pilates will help you increase joint mobility while strengthening the muscles that support the joints.

- Your spine has three natural curves in it: the cervical curve, a slight forward curve at the top of the spine (i.e., the neck); the thoracic curve, a slight backward curve in the upper back; and the lumbar curve, a slight forward curve at the lower back. Pilates exercises help strengthen the back and spine, while keeping these three curves in alignment. (See spine illustration on page 48.)

(Source: American Physical Therapy Association)

THE SPINE

Figure 5.2

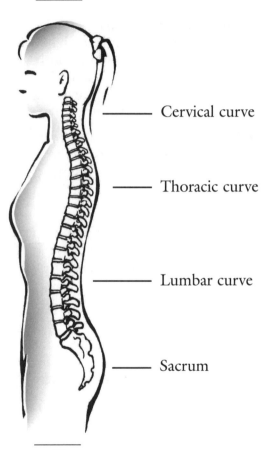

Cervical curve

Thoracic curve

Lumbar curve

Sacrum

Practicing Pilates will help you identify which muscles to use for specific movements. You'll realize as soon as you start the work that the muscles that are the hardest to train are the muscles that haven't been doing their job.

FAB ABS

One of the key elements of good posture is having strong abdominal muscles that support the spine and pelvis. As you read earlier in this book, your core is the center of power, and by developing this area, you'll gain strength, control, and stability in your trunk that will positively effect all of your movements.

There are four abdominal muscles that are layered around the front, back, and sides of the trunk between the rib cage and pelvis, criss-crossing each other in different directions. While they all have specific functions, they also all work together to maintain posture and initiate movements. (See location of abdominal muscles on page 50.)

ABDOMINAL MUSCLES

Figure 5.3

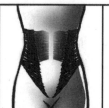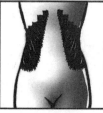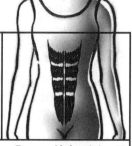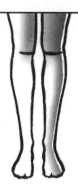

| Transversus Abdominis | Internal Oblique | External Oblique | Rectus Abdominis |

The transversus abdominis is the deepest layer, and wraps horizontally around the back and sides of the torso. Contracting this muscle pulls in the belly. To feel this muscle, place your hands on your sides and cough.

The next layer, the internal oblique, lies between the pelvis and ribs on the sides of the trunk. Although these muscle fibers run in various directions, they are primarily oriented in a diagonal direction, running forward and up from the pelvis. These muscles are used in bending the trunk sideways and forwards.

The external obliques lie on top of the internal obliques, between the pelvis and the middle of the rib cage, and are primarily oriented in a diagonal direction, running forward and down from the ribs. Contracting either or both layers of oblique muscles flattens the stomach area and helps bend the trunk forward. Oblique muscles also work together to rotate the trunk.

You're probably most familiar with the top layer of the abdominals, the rectus abdominis, which runs vertically from the pubic bone to the sternum. When people talk about "six-pack abs" or "a washboard stomach," they're referring to the rectus abdominis.

Pilates helps you work all of these muscles to develop greater core strength. It's also a great way to flatten your stomach and slim your waist. The exercises do their part to increase strength and length in the body, but changing your body shape requires more than practicing Pilates a few times a week. If you want people to see your fab abs, you also have to burn off the fat covering those muscles by following an aerobic training program and a low-fat diet.

ALIGN THE SPINE

Maintaining spinal and pelvic alignment is an important element of good posture. As you read earlier in this chapter, the spine has three natural curves. Correct alignment of these three curves helps the spine function optimally.

Pelvic position can also affect spinal alignment and posture. Physical therapists often use the term "neutral position" or "neutral spine" to describe the pelvis and spine when they are correctly aligned. (Note: Neutral position and neutral spine are not Pilates concepts.)

Try the following postural exercise to find out what it feels like to have your pelvis and spine in neutral position. This exercise should be performed slowly and gently. (See illustration below.)

NEUTRAL POSITION EXERCISE
Figure 5.4

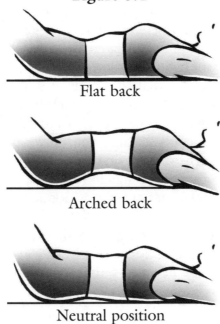

Flat back

Arched back

Neutral position

Health Note: This is a relatively simple exercise, but if you have back pain, injuries, or other health conditions, do not attempt the exercise unless supervised by a physical therapist or a certified Pilates instructor.

1. Lie on your back on the floor or on a mat.
2. Place your hand between your lower back and the floor; you should have a natural curve there.
3. Remove your hand and use your abdominal muscles to tilt your pelvis in so that the small of your back presses flat against the floor and your stomach flattens.
4. Now use your lower back muscles to tilt your pelvis in the opposite direction, arching your lower back.
5. Finally, return to your first position in Step 2, which is neutral position, and engage your abdominal muscles but keep your pelvis in neutral position.

You can try this same exercise with your neck. Lie on the floor and tilt your head back, slowly and gently, raising your chin in the air. This position puts an exaggerated arch in the neck.

Figure 5.5

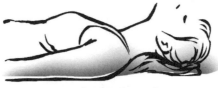

Arched neck

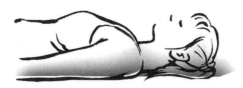

Neutral position

To achieve neutral position, you need to have a straight neck (there will still be a small natural curve so your neck will not flatten against the floor), with your chin parallel to the floor or slightly tilted forward. Your eyes should look straight up to the ceiling (see illustration on page 55). If you have trouble finding neutral position in these exercises, ask a physical therapist or a Pilates or yoga instructor to walk you through them.

6 | Pilatespeak

Sometimes the jargon and descriptions used in exercise books and classes can be confusing and intimidating. That's why I've listed and defined in this chapter several expressions and terms that you might hear in a typical Pilates class. If you can become familiar with some of the major guidelines and vocabulary before you begin, you'll be able to spend more energy concentrating on the exercises.

I've also included definitions for some of the terms used in this book, especially descriptions used in the exercise instructions in Chapter 8. In order to help you develop greater awareness of your body and of how different muscles are used to make movements, I've tried where appropriate to use a movement, visual image, or sensation rather than a common phrase or instruction. For example, instead of using "navel to spine," a common Pilates instruction, I've written "pull your abs toward your spine (from the pubic bone to the sternum)" so that you understand which muscle to use and where it's located.

Understanding individual muscles, positions, and movements will help you isolate and integrate your muscles for a more balanced body. Pilates is not just an exercise method; it's also an educational system that can help you become more in tune with your body.

TERMS	DEFINITIONS
B line	The B Line is one of the key elements of good posture. You need to maintain a straight line (B line), parallel to the floor, from the top of one hip bone to the other. Then a few inches below the belly button, engage your lower abdominal muscles.

Box, the

A term used by Pilates instructors to describe correct alignment. The box is formed by the horizontal lines of the hips and shoulders and the vertical lines between the hips and shoulders. While exercising, you want to keep your shoulders in line with your hips.

C curve

The C curve describes the position of the lower back when doing some Pilates exercises, like Spine Stretch. As you pull your abdominal muscles in and up towards the spine, you also lift out of your hips, stretching your spine and extending through the head so that your form a C curve with your lower back (see Scoop).

Contrology

The original name of Joseph Pilates' exercise method, now called "Pilates." He promoted his work as a method to restore good posture, balance, and strength without building bulky muscles.

Engage (engaged, engaging)

To gently contract a muscle during an exercise.

Exercise band

A thin, rubber strap about four inches wide and three to four feet long used in physical therapy and other exercises.

Extend

Extend is used in the exercise instructions to mean reach or stretch a limb. For example, in Single Leg Stretch, when you straighten and lengthen one leg, leading with your heel, you are extending that leg.

Extension

An anatomical term used to describe backward bending, usually of the spine.

Flexion

To bend forward. Many of the exercises in this book, like The Hundred, The Roll-Up, and Spine Stretch, involve forward flexion of the spine.

Functional exercise

Exercises that prepare the body for real-life functional movements like sitting, standing, walking, running, playing tennis, etc. Pilates is a functional exercise because it conditions core muscles, limbs, and joints in an integrated way, improving alignment, building overall body strength, and resulting in more efficient movement.

Hip flexors

The muscles that run vertically through the crease where your leg and pelvis meet. These muscles help move the leg.

Mind-body connection

Pilates referred to his exercise system as "complete coordination of body, mind, and spirit." One goal in Pilates is to perform the exercises with mindfulness, paying full attention to your movements and breathing, to better integrate the mind and body.

Navel to spine

This term is used in many books and classes to describe a key movement in Pilates exercises. When performing exercises, you need to use the abdominal muscles to control your movement and to protect the lower back by stabilizing and supporting the spine. To achieve this support, you pull your rectus abdominis muscle up and in toward your spine, from the pubic bone to the sternum. See "Pull abs up and in."

Neuromuscular patterning

Throughout your life, movements, gravity, and emotions all contribute to the way your nervous system and muscles function. Over time patterns get set in the body—some healthy, some that prevent the body from functioning optimally. Through exercises like Pilates and yoga, and through some types of deep tissue body work like Soma or Hellerwork, unhealthy patterns can be corrected or "repatterned" to promote healthier tissues.

Neutral spine

A key element of good posture. When the spine is in neutral position that means it is in optimal alignment. Holding the body in this position requires less energy and allows the most free and efficient movement. See page 52 for a description of how to find neutral spine.

Powerhouse, the This term describes the core area on which Pilates exercises are focused: abdominal muscles, lower back muscles, gluteus maximus muscles. This area falls within the box (page 59). The goal is to strengthen and integrate these muscles. Some instructors call this area "the girdle of strength."

Prone Lying on your stomach.

Pull abs up and in This is a direction used in the exercise instructions of this book to describe the correct position of the abdominal muscles during exercise. It is also called "navel to spine." You need to lengthen the rectus abdominis muscle as if energy was traveling up and out through the top of the muscle and down and out through the bottom of the muscle at the same time that you pull the muscle down against your spine, from pubic bone to sternum. This movement helps protect the lower back by supporting the spine. See "Navel to spine."

Range of movement

The range in which you can move a body part around a joint without other body parts aiding in the movement. For example, in Single Leg Circle, your range of movement would be the size of the circle you can make with your raised leg without recruiting other muscles to help move the leg. As you become stronger and more flexible in the joints and develop greater control, you can increase the range of movement. Also referred to as range of motion.

Roll up, roll down the vertebrae

Your spine was never meant to be straight as a rod. One goal of Pilates is to exercise the spine in order to maintain its natural curves and flexibility. Rolling up means that when you raise your torso off the floor from a supine position (controlling the movement with your abs), you want to articulate your spine, allowing each vertebra to stack on top of the one beneath it until you reach a sitting position. Lift the top of your neck first, and slowly peel each vertebra off the floor. If you continue to move the torso forward, engaging abs, you give the spine a good stretch. Rolling down means that from a seated position, you articulate the spine as you did rolling up—placing one vertebra against the floor from tailbone to the top of the spine.

Rotation

Movement around an axis. For example, twisting the torso from side to side, as in Criss Cross.

Scooped, Scoop

Scooping refers to the movement and held position of your abdominals as you pull them up and in toward your spine. Imagine an ice cream scoop scooping up your abdomen, from pubic bone to sternum, hollowing out your stomach.

Sit bones

Instructors use this expression to describe two bony prominences at the bottom of the pelvis. When the pelvis is in neutral position, you should be able to feel the "sit bone" in each buttock making contact with the floor.

Sternum

Breast bone.

Supine

Lying on your back.

7 | Getting Started

A PERSONAL PLAN

The best way to learn about Pilates is to work privately with a qualified, certified Pilates instructor. Your instructor will help you become more aware of the different muscles in your body and how to use them to perform the movements correctly. Practicing correct form in your exercises is the key to benefiting from Pilates.

If the cost of private lessons is prohibitive for you, there are other options. You could take semi-private lessons or attend group mat classes. If you choose to take mat classes, try to find a small class with an instructor who explains the correct form for each exercise. People with injuries or health problems should seek private instruction.

Reading this book will also help you prepare by serving as an at-home practice guide, as well as introducing you to the philosophies, guidelines, and vocabulary behind Pilates.

After four or five sessions you'll have a basic understanding of form and intent, and you'll be ready to practice on your own at home. You might also choose to continue private sessions and/or join a group mat class.

What to Expect

If you have not exercised in a long time, your instructor may start you off on the Pilates machines, which support the body through the movements, making it easier for you to practice the exercises. If you are in good shape, you may start off with mat exercises or a combination of machine and mat exercises.

Before you begin, you'll be asked to fill out a health questionnaire that will help your instructor design a program that fits your individual needs and/or limitations. During the session your instructor will talk you through the exercises, touching you when necessary to help you adjust a position.

Don't be afraid to ask questions or to stop the work if you feel any pain or discomfort. Pilates is not about mindlessly following instructions but about learning, change, and growth.

Health Note: As always, consult with your physician before beginning an exercise program. If you have a medical condition, injury, or any other health concerns, share this information with your instructor so that she can consider this when designing your routine.

Your Goals

What do you want to achieve through Pilates? Clarifying your needs and goals before you begin will help you focus. Maybe you want to improve your posture or add more power to your tennis game. Maybe you're simply in an exercise rut and curious to try something new. Share your goals, concerns, and fears with your instructor so that she can guide and support you on this journey. (There are great female and male Pilates teachers; I've used "she" through this chapter for simplicity and consistency.)

PREGNANCY AND PILATES

Pilates is an excellent exercise for preparing the body for pregnancy because it strengthens the abdominal muscles and pelvic floor. Many women who practice Pilates continue to do so during pregnancy. If you have been practicing Pilates before your pregnancy, work with your doctor and Pilates instructor to design a pre- and post-natal plan. If you have not exercised in a long time, or become pregnant shortly after starting Pilates, it is probably best to wait until you've recovered from the birth before beginning or continuing the work.

HOW TO SELECT A TEACHER

The quality of your instruction can make all the difference in how much you benefit from the work and how much you enjoy the exercise.

While there is no uniform training and certification standard nationwide, there are several quality training programs available. A good program, for example, lasts about nine months to a year and includes workshops, student teaching, and testing. Students complete hundreds of hours of training by the time the program ends.

Qualities to look for when selecting a Pilates instructor:

- **Experience** An instructor with at least three years of teaching experience, someone who regularly practices Pilates as well as teaches it. Ask your instructor to explain the different results her other clients have achieved by working with her.

- **Certification** Your instructor should have completed a rigorous training and certification program, lasting nine to twelve months. Weekend Pilates training seminars do not provide sufficient training for Pilates instruction.

- **Knowledge** An instructor who has completed coursework and testing on anatomy, movement, CPR, and the Pilates method. Ask your instructor if she sharpens her skills with continuing education.

- **Safety** Your instructor should have a deep understanding of how the body responds to exercise, how to modify exercises to accommodate the individual needs of clients, and how to lead you through your routine safely.

- **Patience & Understanding** You should feel that your instructor is focused on you and attuned to your needs, limitations, and energy levels. A good instructor should be patient with you and interested in your overall health.

Some instructors are trained in rehabilitative Pilates and may even practice in a physical therapy office. Others may come from a dance or movement background and be more fitness-focused. Like any other exercise, you may need to shop around to find an instructor who best fits your needs.

PILATES VS. PILATES-BASED EXERCISE

Like many other exercise forms or health practices, there is some confusion, debate, and division in the Pilates world. At the heart of the debate is the meaning of "true Pilates."

Some Pilates instructors believe that in order to benefit from the exercises, you must follow exactly Joseph Pilates' teachings and methods. Other instructors believe that there is room for adaptations.

The debate peaked in the fall of 2000, when a court decided that the name "Pilates" could not be trademarked. Now, Pilates is a generic word like yoga, and anyone who wants to call their exercise Pilates can do so. For this reason, you must always ask about credentials and training to make sure the instruction you receive is accurate and safe. Hopefully, this resolution will bring more integration and standardization nationwide. Currently, a national association of Pilates professionals is being formed.

Although Pilates is a strict discipline, with a designated program to follow, any teacher you work with will have her own style based on her experience and interpretation of the work. The important thing is to work with someone who understands how the body functions so that she can guide you through your exercises safely and correctly, helping you gain maximum benefits.

Classes that are advertised as "Pilates-based" may not be true Pilates nor taught by a certified Pilates instructor. Always ask about credentials.

Class Offerings and Cost

Pilates studios offer a variety of classes and instruction, and the prices may vary from place to place. Expect to pay from $50–75/hour for a private session; $25–40/hour for a semi-private (2–3 people) session; and $10–15/hour for a group mat class. When you call to sign up for a class, you can ask about class size (the smaller, the better), instructor qualifications, what to wear, or any other questions you have. Some studios will let you observe a class before signing up for it. Also ask if the instructor provides any individual attention during class to help you know if you are doing the exercises correctly.

You may also want to visit the studio before you sign up for a class so that you can get a feel for the space. Look around the studio and pay attention to the energy of the room. Do you feel comfortable there? Is the studio roomy and airy? Is the tone of the classes inviting? Are the machines clean and in good condition? You want to make sure that your experience is as comfortable as possible.

One of the first things I hear from people when I talk about Pilates is "it sounds great, but I can't afford it." I agree that $50–60 for a private session is a lot of money to most of us, but I also think that money spent on learning how to take care of your body is the best investment you can make. In the long run, the price of the four or five introductory sessions you'll need to get started will still be less than the cost of a doctor's appointment or joining a gym. And once you've learned the basic form, you can practice Pilates for the rest of your life—for free!

THE MACHINES

The focus of this book is on Pilates mat work, but you may want to try exercising on Pilates machines, as well. Basically, many of the movements and exercises that you do on the mat can be done on the machines under the supervision of a Pilates instructor.

Some people who are new to exercise might have an easier time learning the fundamentals on the machines because the machines help support the body's weight during exercise, making it a little bit easier to perform the required movements. Others are more comfortable beginning with mat exercises. A qualified Pilates instructor can help you decide on which aspect of the work you want to focus.

Just as Pilates exercises can be modified and adapted to suit individual needs, Pilates machines are adjustable to suit beginners and advanced students. The machines and apparatuses you'll see most at studios include The Cadillac, The Reformer, The Barrels, The Chair, and The Magic Circle.

Pilates machines are some of the scariest looking contraptions I've ever seen—but don't let that dissuade you from trying them. The first time I saw The Cadillac, I wasn't sure if it was a medieval torture machine or some kind of suspended gynecological exam table. Thankfully, it was neither, and I found it easy to use with a bit of practice.

The Cadillac is a wooden table with a padded top that stands about three feet high. Metal poles rise up four to five feet from each table leg, and connect at the ends of the poles to a rectangular frame, also made of metal poles. It looks like a canopy bed without the canopy. Springs attached to wooden bars (they look like trapezes) hang down from the canopy poles at each end of the table, and padded ankle cuffs hang down from the poles above the sides of the table.

The Reformer is also a wooden-framed table, standing only a foot or so off of the floor, with a padded top that can slide back and forth along the frame. Both The Cadillac and The Reformer are similar to weight machines (although they allow much more range of motion), but use springs instead of weights to create resistance. Many of the same stretching and strengthening exercises practiced on the mat can be done on these machines, as well as additional exercises designed specifically for machine work.

The Chair and The Barrels are both box-like, padded wooden props used in stretching and strengthening exercises. The Magic Circle, a large plastic circle about sixteen inches in diameter, is used to provide resistance when strengthening the arms, legs, abs, and chest.

You can purchase Pilates equipment for home use and/or use the machines at a Pilates studio during a private, semi-private, or group class. If you want more information about Pilates equipment, see the resource list at the back of the book.

What to Wear

You can wear the same things you usually wear to exercise—comfortable exercise clothing like a T-shirt and shorts (or sweatpants). Some instructors prefer that you wear snugly-fitting clothes so that they can clearly see your body position. Pilates is done without shoes, although you can keep your socks on for most exercises. When standing or using some machines, you'll want to remove your socks.

Practicing at Home

All you need to practice Pilates at home is a little bit of floor space. If you're practicing on uncarpeted floors, you'll want to lie on a thick mat or towel. It's not necessary to spend a lot of money or buy a special Pilates mat. Foam camping mats (½" to 1" thick) will do the job. If you practice on thick carpeting, you may not need an exercise mat.

How often you practice or for how long depends on your unique goals, body type, fitness level, and physical limitations, if any. If you have never exercised before, or haven't exercised in a long time, you may only be able to do five or ten minutes of Pilates exercises when you first begin. That's okay. Remember that Pilates is about quality, not quantity.

It's important to set aside the time to practice at least twice a week, preferably three or four times a week. Find a time of day that works for you so that you can establish a regular routine. Wait at least an hour after eating a light meal before practicing Pilates, longer after a heavy meal.

Some instructors recommend working up to a one-hour workout three to five times a week. You may find that a thirty- to forty-five-minute workout fits in better with your schedule. In *Return to Life*, Pilates recommends practicing four times a week in order to see changes in your body within three months. Your instructor can start you off on a routine designed for your fitness level and goals that you can practice on your own.

Health Note: Do not exercise if you are sick or feeling very fatigued.

SAMPLE WORKOUTS

The exercises in this book are meant to be followed in order. Most people will have a hard time completing the entire series in one workout. For that reason, I've broken down the list into smaller segments to show you how to gradually increase the length and intensity of your practice.

The stages and times indicated are not written in stone, but are merely guidelines to help you see how you might plan your workouts. You might spend weeks working up to five exercises, or you might be able to complete ten exercises the first time you try. Remember, don't judge yourself by other people's progress or bodies. Progress at your own pace.

Perform the exercises slowly and deliberately. Work at the same pace you would if you were stretching, but don't go so slowly that you lose the rhythm and flow of your movements. As you become more proficient, pick up the pace a little bit, moving swiftly from one exercise to the next. Finally, if you can only exercise for a few minutes, it's better to try a few exercises than repeat one exercise.

- **5–15 minutes**   Start at the beginning of the list (on page 91); try to do up to four or five exercises.

- **15–20 minutes**   Start at the beginning of the list; try to do five to ten exercises.

- **20–30 minutes**   Start at the beginning of the list; try to do ten to fifteen exercises.

- **30–45 minutes**   Start at the beginning of the list; try to do two sets of each exercise.

- **45–60 minutes**   Start at the beginning of the list; try to do three sets of each exercise.

8 | The Mat Exercises

Many consider Pilates mat exercises to be the core of Joseph Pilates' work. This series of exercises, performed in a specific sequence, was designed to help people strengthen and stretch their bodies, regain correct movement and posture, and increase mind-body awareness. Because these exercises can be done anywhere by anyone, they are the most accessible aspect of the Pilates method.

Of Pilates' original thirty-four core mat exercises, I have included in this book fifteen that are appropriate for beginning and intermediate level students, omitting advanced exercises and others that could pose an injury risk if not performed correctly.

The Mat Exercises

If you think that fifteen exercises doesn't sound like much to do, you'll soon realize as you get into the work that practicing and mastering these exercises will keep you plenty busy, whether you want to do a ten-minute or an hour-long workout. The illustrations may make Pilates look easy, but if you perform the exercises correctly, they will be challenging.

Even the basic exercises are challenging because you'll be using muscles that you probably haven't used before. Many of the exercises include modifications that give you the option to decrease and/or increase difficulty. Remember, you're striving for quality movements, not endless repetitions.

Before reading the instructions, you may want to review the terms in Pilatespeak and the muscle groups on the chart on page 11.

All of the exercise instructions, and the sequence, were selected with the guidance of a certified Pilates instructor with more than ten years of teaching experience. The exercises were also reviewed for accuracy and safety by two additional Pilates instructors.

Some of the exercises or their modifications may be slightly different from exercises you've learned in class. You'll notice after working with different instructors that everyone interprets and teaches according to her own style.

How to Follow the Instructions

After you have read the first seven chapters of this book, read through all of the exercise instructions and tips slowly to become more familiar with the movements you'll be making. Then, when you're ready to begin, you can reread each exercise before you practice it. I've tried to keep the instructions free of Pilates jargon, although I have defined some of that jargon in Chapter 6 so that you won't be lost if you go to a Pilates class.

You'll notice that all of the exercises follow the same easy-to-follow format, which includes:

- *Name of the exercise.*
- *Benefits* that can be gained by practicing the exercise correctly and regularly.
- *Instructions* that describe how to perform the exercise.
- *Tips and modification* that give more information about form and movement.

- *Cautions* about health concerns or injuries that may be aggravated by performing the exercise.
- *Rating* that indicates a beginning (I) or intermediate (II) level exercise.
- *Illustrations* that reflect the essence of each exercise. (Follow the written instructions; use the illustrations as a visual guide only.)

Health Note: Please note that the cautions and rating categories are to be used as general guidelines. As mentioned on page 69, consult a physician before starting a new exercise routine. If you have any health conditions or concerns, discuss them with your doctor. If you have osteoporosis, do not do any of the forward bending exercises. Taking a few Pilates classes before you begin is recommended to learn correct form.

Depending on your experience, body type, health, and fitness level, you may find exercises rated I to be just as challenging as exercises rated II. If an exercise feels too difficult, move on to the next one. Don't continue if you feel pain, discomfort, dizziness, or any other uncomfortable sensation.

TIPS TO KEEP YOU ON TRACK

These tips are based on the eight guidelines outlined in Chapter 4.

Go with the Flow

The instructions may seem long at first glance, but as you read them closely you'll see that they, along with the tips and modifications, contain information about all the different areas of your body that need to work together to practice the exercise in correct form. The more you practice, the easier it will be to integrate all of the information in your head and body so that you can perform the exercises fluidly. Think of each exercise as a dance that your body moves through with grace and precision.

Length and Strength

As you perform the movements of each exercise, remember to feel the stretch whenever you extend your spine or limbs. Maintain your strength and stability by keeping your core muscles engaged (i.e., feel your abs pulling in toward your spine and wrapping around your waist). Visualize long limbs, and length between your hips and ribs, shoulders and ears.

Isolate and Integrate

Concentrate on your movements so that you can isolate areas of the body when necessary and integrate different muscles during your movements to increase stability and strength.

Align and Assign

Remember to maintain correct alignment when performing the exercises. Keep your shoulders parallel to hips, knees and ankles in line with hips, and shoulders down and away from ears. Also, assign the correct muscles to perform specific movements. Don't rely on momentum or old patterns to get you through; the purpose is to retrain muscles to function in optimal patterning.

Keep Breathing

Some of the breathing instructions in this book may differ from what you might learn in a class. Breathing techniques can vary from instructor to instructor. If you find it too difficult to coordinate your movements with the breath, simply continue to breathe in and out as you do the exercise. Do not hold your breath. With practice, you'll be able to begin integrating the breathing with your movements.

As a general rule, breathe through your nose. Inhale when you open or extend the body, and exhale as you close the body or bend forward. Use your breath to aid your movement.

Patience and Persistence

It may take a while for you to get used to these exercises, and a bit longer to understand them completely. Hang in there, and don't be too hard on yourself. Meanwhile, enjoy learning more about your body and training it to move with more strength, grace, and flexibility. Like any new exercise, there will be a learning curve, and like any goal you want to achieve, you need to persevere to succeed. Imagine how you'll feel when you start to see the benefits of your hard work.

A Note About Abs

When the instructions tell you to pull your abs up and in toward your spine, it means activate and lengthen your abdominal muscles. This movement helps protect the spine and lower back during exercise. Some Pilates instructors use the term "navel to spine" to describe this movement.

You probably won't be able to feel the deepest layers of your abdominal muscles as you pull your abs up and in, but they do help make that movement happen. The deepest abdominal layers run horizontally around your waist and, when contracted, pull in toward the spine like the top of a drawstring bag when it's cinched together.

The top layer of the abdominal muscles is the rectus abdominis, which runs vertically from your pubic bone to your rib cage. You will be able to feel that muscle when you pull it up and in toward your spine. Basically, pulling your abs in brings the abs closer to your spine, and pulling them up at the same time helps lengthen the muscle. (Don't hold your breath during this movement, but exhale as you pull in your abs.) Exercising a muscle when it's lengthened helps develop long, lean, functional muscles.

Visualize energy moving from the center of the rectus abdominis muscle and out each end to help you create more length. You may find this concept difficult at first, but it will make more sense the more you practice. Look at the illustrations on page 50 to help you identify the location of the abdominal muscles.

A Note About Glutes

Some Pilates instructors emphasize "engaging the thighs and buttocks" during certain exercises to help stabilize and support the lower back. Other instructors seem to apply this direction on an individual basis.

When the exercise instructions direct you to engage your thighs and buttocks, they don't mean simply clenching your buttocks together. Instead, try to visualize the area at the top of the back of your leg, where the upper hamstrings and lower gluteal muscles meet. That's the area that you want to activate.

THE EXERCISES

The exercises should be practiced in the following order:

The Hundred
The Roll-Up
Single Leg Circle
Single Leg Stretch
Double Leg Stretch
Criss Cross
Spine Stretch
Saw
Single Leg Kick*
Double Leg Kick*
Spine Twist
Side Kick*
Side Leg Raises*
Swimming*
Child's Pose

Exercises with an asterisk should be followed by Child's Pose, a yoga pose that stretches the back after exercises that extend the spine.

THE HUNDRED

Benefits

Warms up the body in preparation for the rest of the exercises, stimulates lungs and heart, increases circulation, and strengthens abdominal muscles.

Instructions

1. Lie on your back with your arms at your sides, palms down, and your legs together, breathing normally. Before you initiate any movement, inhale slowly.

2. Exhale as you bend your legs and bring your knees to your chest, one at a time. Adjust your legs so that your thighs are perpendicular to the floor and your lower legs are parallel to the floor. In other words, your legs should form a 90° angle. Keep your inner thighs and your ankles pressed together. Inhale.

3. Exhale as you pull your abdominal muscles up and in toward your spine. At the same time slowly curl your head forward, chin toward chest, and raise your upper body off

THE HUNDRED
Figure 8.1

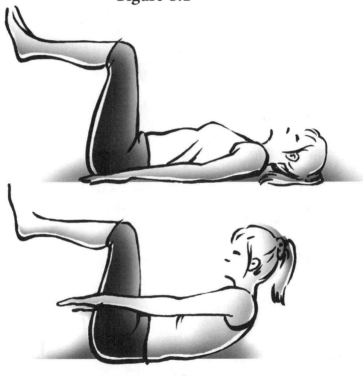

the floor until you feel the base of your shoulder blades touching the floor. Use your abdominal muscles to stabilize your back and to control your movement. Notice that your quads and hip flexors (muscles that activate when you bring your knee to your chest) will contract as you raise your body. Try to relax these muscles so that your abs do most of the work.

As you raise your upper body, keep both arms straight and parallel to the floor. Keep your shoulders down away from your ears, chest relaxed, and arms reaching forward through the fingertips.

4. Inhale for a count of five, then exhale for a count of five while you hold this position. Return to lying on your back by slowly rolling the spine to the floor, vertebra by vertebra.

5. Repeat exercise five to ten times.

Tips and Modifications

- In Step 4, breathe into your back and ribs as you inhale.
- Think of adding length to your ab muscles; visualize energy moving out from each end of the rectus abdominis muscle.

- If this exercise is too difficult, place a pillow under your shoulders and another small pillow on top of that pillow under your head. This will raise the body, making it easier for you to raise yourself up.
- To increase the challenge: Instead of holding your arms in a raised position in Step 4, pump them up and down rapidly (within a small range of motion—4 to 6"—using precision and control) while inhaling for five counts, then exhaling for five.
- To further increase the challenge: Instead of doing the exercise with knees bent, try to do it with your legs straight and at a 45° angle with the floor.
- While your upper body is raised off the floor, continue to pull abs to spine. (Don't let abs push out.)
- Engage inner thigh muscles and buttocks (upper hamstrings/lower glutes) to increase lower back stability.

Caution: If you feel neck tension, rest your head back on the mat.

Rating: I–II

THE ROLL-UP

Benefits

Exercises, stretches, and strengthens the spine, stretches hamstrings, develops core strength, and decompresses the lower back.

Instructions

1. Lie on your back with your arms over your head, palms up, and legs together.

2. Inhale as you raise your arms perpendicular to the body, reaching your fingertips toward the ceiling. Exhale as you pull your abs to your spine and slowly roll up into a sitting position, using your abs to stabilize your back and control movement. Keep your arms extended in front of you, parallel to the floor, reaching forward through the fingertips.

3. Continue exhaling as you roll forward, keeping your abs

THE ROLL-UP
Figure 8.2

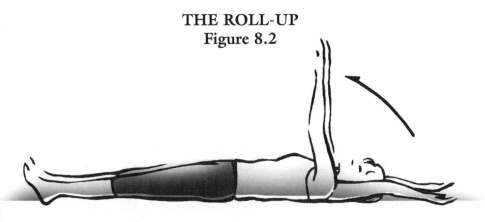

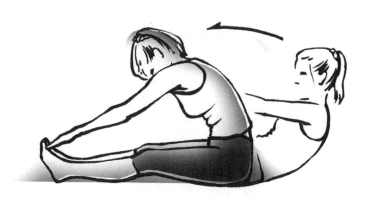

pulled up and in toward your spine, and stretch your torso over your legs, keeping your head between your arms, and reaching past your feet with your hands. Don't let your body collapse over your legs. Keep lifting your torso out of your hips. As you roll forward, reach forward with the top of your head. Try to keep your lower body glued to the floor.

4. Keeping your abs pulled in toward your spine, slowly roll back into a supine position, one vertebra at a time. First, inhale as you raise your body into a seated position, then exhale as you lie back on the mat.

5. Repeat exercise three to five times.

Tips and Modifications

- Use your breath to help you control the movement.
- Engage your inner thighs and buttocks (upper hamstrings/ lower glutes) to help stabilize the lower back. Don't lock knees.
- For more stability, squeeze a small rubber ball or cushion between your knees, and another between your ankles.
- Make sure your chin is dropped towards the chest and that you don't pull with your head or neck when you roll up or down; use your ab muscles to initiate and control movement.

- Keep shoulders down and away from ears, chest relaxed.
- To make this exercise more manageable, you can keep your legs bent, with your feet on the floor, heels about one foot away from buttocks. Keep your feet on the floor throughout the exercise.
- If raising yourself is too difficult, start from an upright seated position, legs bent, feet firmly planted on the floor. Place your right hand under your right thigh, and your left hand under your left thigh. Using your abs to stabilize and control the movement, slowly roll your body toward the floor, vertebra by vertebra, from tailbone to head, until your arms are straight and parallel to the floor. (You'll be leaning back, but most of your back will not touch the floor.) Roll back up to a seated position using your abs to control the movement.
- You can also use an exercise band to modify the exercise. Begin from a seated position, loop an exercise band around your feet, and hold on to the band as you lower yourself to the floor, vertebra by vertebra.

Cautions: If you feel tension in your neck, lie back down on the mat. Be careful if you have lower back pain.

Rating: I

SINGLE LEG CIRCLE

Benefits

Strengthens and increases mobility in the hip joints, stretches hamstrings, inner thighs (adductor muscles), and outer thighs (abductor muscles and iliotibial band).

Instructions

1. Lie on your back with your arms at your sides, palms down, legs together. Inhale before initiating any movement.

2. As you exhale, pull your abs up and in toward your spine to stabilize your lower back, and bring your right knee to your chest. Then raise your right leg in the air, perpendicular to the floor, keeping your leg straight. If you can't keep your raised leg straight, it's okay to bend the knee a little bit. Rotate your raised leg slightly so that your heel points toward your stable leg and your toes point away from the right side of your body.

SINGLE LEG CIRCLE
Figure 8.3

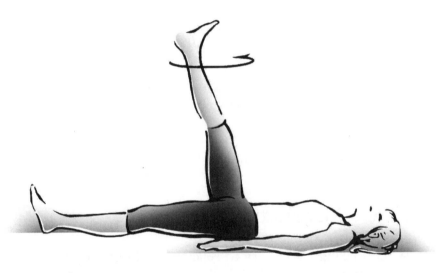

3. Keep your body pressed to the floor, especially the backs of your hips. Imagine that your pelvis is holding a large bowl of water—your goal is to perform the exercise without spilling any water. In other words, you don't want

the bowl moving from side to side or up and down. The more stable your lower body is, the more you can isolate the adductor muscles, target the hip joint, and have free range of motion in your hips.

4. Breathe normally, making a small circle in the air with your right foot in a clockwise direction. Repeat for five more circles. Then do six circles in the opposite direction. Then bring your right knee back to your chest and then to the floor.

5. Repeat exercise six times with left leg raised.

Tips and Modifications

- When making circles, try to relax your hip flexors (the muscles in front of your hips). Rely on your inner thigh muscles to help rotate the leg.
- Be careful not to let your raised leg drop too low or your back arch off the mat. Keep lower back pressed to the floor and abs engaged.

- As you become more proficient, you can make bigger circles as long as the movement is precise and controlled.
- This can be a difficult exercise to do, especially first thing in the morning when your hamstrings are tight. If making circles with a raised leg is too difficult, loop an exercise band around the foot of your straightened leg, holding both ends in one hand to help control the circles. Or, bend your raised leg to a 90° angle (calf parallel to floor) and make circles with your bent leg. Or, keep your raised leg straight and bend your supporting leg, pressing into the floor with your foot.

Caution: Be careful if you have lower back pain or hip problems.

Rating: I

SINGLE LEG STRETCH

Benefits

Stretches and strengthens legs and lower back, strengthens abdominal muscles, and increases coordination and hip- and knee-joint mobility.

Instructions

1. Lie on your back with your arms at your sides, palms down, legs together. Before you initiate any movement, inhale slowly.

2. Exhale as you pull your abs up and in toward your spine, raise your upper body off the floor as you roll your head forward, chin toward chest, until you feel the base of your shoulder blades touching the floor. At the same time, pull your knees into your chest, one at a time. Place your hands on your legs, just below the knees.

SINGLE LEG STRETCH
Figure 8.4

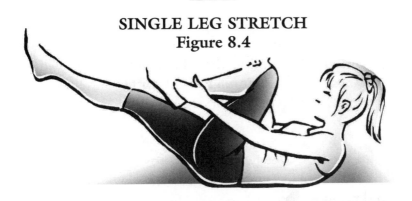

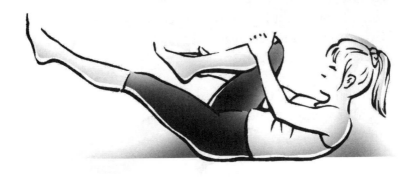

3. As you inhale place your right hand on your left knee and your left hand on the outside of your left leg midway between your calf and ankle. This hand position will help you keep your leg in alignment with your hips as you move. Extend your right leg at a 45° angle with the floor.

4. As you exhale slowly, switch the positions of your legs so that you extend your left leg at a 45° angle with the floor and bring your right knee toward your chest. You will also switch the positions of your hands so that your left hand is on your right knee and your right hand is on the outside of your right leg midway between your calf and ankle. Continue pulling abs toward spine, and keep your lower back pressed flat against the floor.

5. Continue doing the exercise, inhaling for one full movement (extend leg and retract it), then exhaling for one full movement. Repeat five to ten times.

Tips and Modifications

- Keep your upper body still; only your arms and legs should be moving.
- Keep your chest open, shoulders in line, hip flexors relaxed, shoulders away from ears, and elbows off the floor. Your torso should not be twisting during leg movement.
- Coordinate movement with breath, inhaling through nose and exhaling through mouth.

Cautions: If you have bad knees, try placing your right hand under your thigh and your left hand under your knee for more support in Step 3. If you experience any neck pain, rest your head on a small pillow or lie back down on the mat.

Rating: I

DOUBLE LEG STRETCH

Benefits

Strengthens and stretches legs, strengthens abdominal muscles, stretches arms, increases coordination, and mobilizes shoulder joints.

Instructions

1. Lie on your back with your arms at your sides, palms down, legs together. Before initiating movement, inhale slowly.

2. Exhale as you pull your abs up and in toward your spine, raise your upper body off the floor as you roll your head forward, chin toward chest. At the same time, pull your knees into your chest and then place your hands on your legs, just below the knees.

3. As you inhale slowly, extend your legs to a 45°–60° angle, and raise your arms up in the air and reach behind your

**DOUBLE LEG
STRETCH
Figure 8.5**

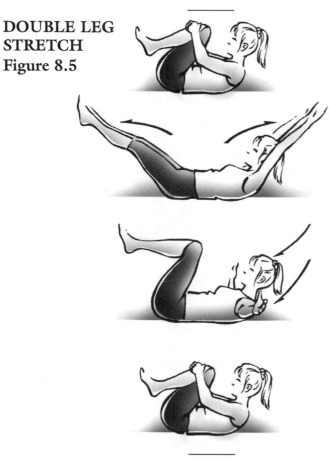

head until your arms line up with your ears. Keep your abs pulled to your spine and visualize energy moving out your fingertips and toes as you extend your arms and legs. Also visualize your rectus abdominis muscles lengthening.

4. As you exhale slowly, sweep your arms from their extended position away from the body until they are forming a straight line perpendicular to the body. As you continue sweeping your arms forward, pull your knees back into your chest and place your hands on your legs, just below the knees. Maintain abs to spine.

5. Repeat exercise five to ten times.

Tips and Modifications

- Keep your back on the mat throughout the movement. Your upper body should remain still, chest open and relaxed.
- As you extend your legs, engaging your inner thighs and buttocks (upper hamstrings/lower glutes) will keep your legs to-

gether. You don't want your legs straying beyond the line between shoulder and hip when you extend.

- Maintain the position of your head and neck when you reach your arms over your head and throughout the movement. Don't let your head drop back. If you need more support, you can place a cushion or pillow under your shoulders and head.
- Remember to keep reaching through the fingertips and toes.

Caution: Be careful if you have lower back problems. If you feel pain, stop.

Rating: I

CRISS CROSS

Benefits

Strengthens abdominal muscles, working them diagonally to strengthen obliques, creates length in torso, and improves coordination and balance.

Instructions

1. Lie on your back with your fingertips at the sides of your head, legs together. Inhale before initiating any movement.

2. Exhale as you pull your abs toward your spine to stabilize your body, bring your right knee to your chest, and raise your extended left leg to a 45° angle. At the same time slowly curl your head forward, chin toward chest, and raise your upper body off the floor until you feel the base of your shoulder blades against the floor. Do not pull forward with the head; raise the body using your abs. Inhale, then continue breathing normally.

CRISS CROSS
Figure 8.6

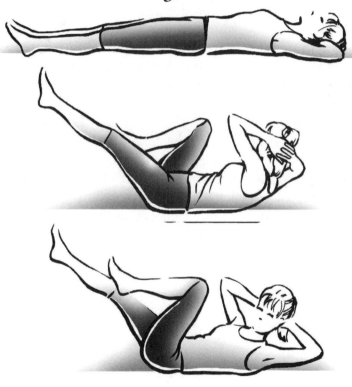

3. Rotate your upper torso to the right, keeping your elbows wide and your chest open and reaching toward your right knee with your left shoulder as you look past your right elbow. (Touching your knee with your elbow or shoulder is not the goal.) Lowering your chin a bit toward your chest will help you as you turn your head. Do not lead the movement with elbow or shoulder, but lift and twist out of your waist.

4. Rotate your body back to the center as you switch leg positions, extending your right leg to a 45° angle and bringing your left knee toward your chest. Reach toward the inside of your left knee with the right shoulder. You can lower the upper body a bit as you switch leg positions, but continue to keep the shoulder blades off the floor, abs engaged, and the backs of your hips pressed to the mat. Keep your torso as still as possible, and try not to let your body move from side to side.

5. Repeat sequence three to five times.

Tips and Modifications

- Do not use your arms to raise your body or to pull your head forward. This could put strain on the neck. Remember to use your abs to initiate and control movement; do not lead the twisting movement with your elbows. Unless you are incredibly flexible and strong, you will not be able to touch your elbow to your knee. Remember to extend through your elbows throughout the exercise, keeping elbows in line with your ears. Looking past your elbow when you twist the torso will help engage the deeper layers of your abdominal muscles.
- You want to lengthen through the obliques (the sides of your torso) in this exercise, so as you twist the torso to one side, feel the extension in the opposite side of the body. Basically, as one side contracts, the other side lengthens, working the abs diagonally.
- Feel the extension in your legs as you reach the toes of your extended leg toward the opposite wall. Engaging your inner thighs and keeping your knees together will help you keep your legs in line with your hips. Keep the backs of your hips firmly planted to the floor. And don't let your extended leg drop.

- Keep chest and neck relaxed. Look straight ahead and do not let your chin fall toward your chest. As you turn to make the trunk twist, lower your chin a bit and look out past the elbow.
- Feel the top of the ab muscles, just below your sternum, engage to help rotate your upper torso. Visualize the rib cage spiraling from side to side around the spine. Twist slowly, and hold the twist as you reach back with your elbow. Exhale completely with the twist, as if you're wringing out the lungs. Remember to lift and twist at your waist; your neck and shoulders should remain relaxed.

Caution: Be careful if you have neck or shoulder problems.

Rating: II

SPINE STRETCH

Benefits

Stretches spine, works deepest layers of abdominal muscles, promotes good posture, stretches hamstrings, and facilitates improved breathing by making rib-cage muscles more supple.

Instructions

1. Sit on the floor with legs extended, feet a bit wider than hip-width apart, and arms extended in front of you, parallel to the floor. Sit tall (on your sit bones) in good posture with abdominal muscles engaged, head held high, shoulders aligned over hips, chest slightly raised, ankles flexed (pressing out through the heels).

2. As you inhale, lift your torso out of your hips, extending your spine as if someone was pulling a string out of the top of your head.

SPINE STRETCH
Figure 8.7

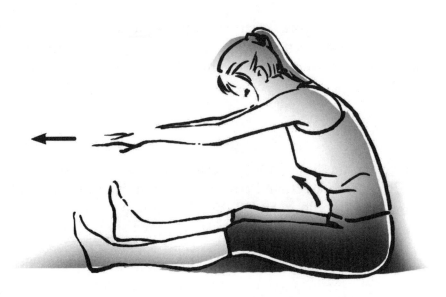

3. As you exhale, still pulling your abs up and in toward your spine, roll your chin forward toward your chest, and continue moving forward, controlling your forward movement with your abs. Remember as you move forward to keep lifting your torso out of your hips and extend through the top of your head, forming a C with your lower back. As you reach forward with your fingertips and the top of your head, visualize that you have a wide towel wrapped around your stomach and someone is standing behind you, pulling on the towel.

4. Continue rolling your body forward over your legs. You want to be extending through your arms as you reach your fingertips forward, as if someone is holding your hands and gently pulling you forward.

5. Reach past your toes, and inhale slowly, breathing into your back and filling your ribs as you slowly return to your original sitting position, rolling back up one vertebra at a time. Exhale.

6. Repeat exercise three to five times.

Tips and Modifications

- If it is difficult for you to sit in this position, try raising your pelvis a bit by sitting on a folded towel or mat.
- If you cannot keep your legs straight, it is okay to bend the knees. Or, place rolled-up towels under your knees for support. Do not lock your knees.
- Make sure that you are pulling your abs up and in toward your spine, and control your movement with your abs. Don't hinge through the hips.
- Remember to extend through the arms, legs, and spine. Engage inner thighs and buttocks (upper hamstrings/lower glutes) to increase stability.
- A simpler version is to sit in the starting position, then as you roll your body forward, keep hands on the floor, fingers pointing toward feet, in between your thighs. As you bend over your legs, slowly move hands forward, maintaining contact with the floor. You won't be able to go as low as in the original exercise, but you will still gain benefits.

Caution: Don't do this exercise if you have osteoporosis.

Rating: I

SAW

Benefits

Stretches hamstrings and strengthens core muscles, facilitates exhaling breath to fully expel air in preparation for full inhalation.

Instructions

1. Sit on the floor with your legs extended, feet a bit wider than hips-width apart, and arms extended at shoulder height to each side of your body, parallel to the floor. Sit tall (on your sit bones) in good posture with abdominal muscles engaged, head held high, shoulders aligned over your hips, and shoulder blades pressed flat against back, chest slightly raised.

2. As you inhale, stretch your spine, extending through the top of your head, as if someone was pulling a string out of

SAW
Figure 8.8

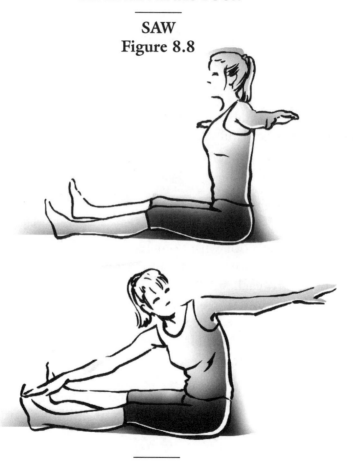

the top of your head, and lift your torso out of your hips. Pull your abs to your spine.

3. As you exhale, twist your torso to the left, controlling the movement with your abs. Keep your legs and buttocks glued to the floor. Feel the extension through your arms as you reach with your fingertips. Lower your body forward over your legs, as you reach your right hand forward so that your right pinkie finger can "saw" your left pinkie toe. Keep extending through the spine.

4. Keeping abs pulled to spine, slowly return to your original upright position as you inhale. Repeat the exercise on the opposite side of the body, then repeat the sequence three to five times.

Tips and Modifications

• If it is difficult for you to sit in this position and keep your legs straight, try raising your pelvis a bit by sitting on a folded towel or mat.

- If you cannot keep your legs straight, it is okay to bend the knees a little bit, or place rolled-up towels under your knees for support.
- Keep your feet flexed, extending through heels.
- Don't move through the hips; you should control the movement with your abs and feel a stretch in your side as you reach for your toe. Try to relax your hip flexors.

Caution: Don't do this exercise if you have osteoporosis, or shoulder, neck, or lower back pain.

Rating: II

SINGLE LEG KICK

Benefits

Stretches quads (fronts of thighs), strengthens hamstrings, and works biceps and triceps.

Instructions

1. Lie on your stomach, with your arms in front of you, forehead resting on your stacked hands (palms to floor). Keep your legs together, toes slightly pointed. Pull your abs to your spine, and press your pubic bone to the floor.

2. Raise your chest off the floor, and prop yourself up with your arms so that your forearms are resting on the floor in front of you, and your hands are in fists, thumb side facing up. Your elbows should be in line with your shoulders (if your lower back feels compacted, move your arms forward a bit to lower your upper body). Keep chest relaxed, shoul-

SINGLE LEG KICK
Figure 8.9

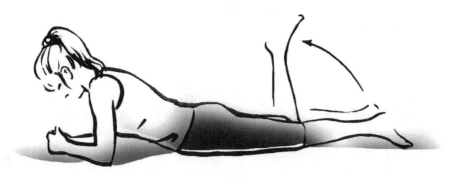

ders down from ears, and look forward, just a few inches past your fists on the floor to keep your neck straight.

3. Keeping your pubic bone pressed to the floor and your abs engaged, bend your right knee, bringing your heel toward your butt. You'll feel this in your hamstrings. Keep toes pointed and knees together. Then lower your right leg to the floor (you'll feel this in your thigh), as you bring your left heel toward your buttock.

4. Continue this sequence five to ten times, inhaling for one set (right leg up and down), exhaling for the next (left leg up and down). Follow this exercise with Child's Pose on page 148.

Tips and Modifications

• To increase the stretch in the back and front of your legs, slightly flex your ankle when you raise your leg, extending through the heel, and slightly point your toes, as you lower your leg.

- To increase the challenge, after raising your heel toward your butt, gently pump your bent leg twice (toward the back of your head) before lowering it.
- Protect your lower back by keeping abs engaged and pubic bone pressed to the floor. Your hips may raise off the floor slightly.

Caution: Don't do this exercise if you have knee problems.

Rating: II

DOUBLE LEG KICK

Benefits

Strengthens and stretches shoulders and midback, works the backs of the legs and buttocks.

Instructions

1. Lie on the floor on your stomach, head resting on right side, legs together. Rest your right hand on your lower back, palm up, and place your left hand, palm up, in your right hand.

2. Pull your abs to your spine and press your hips and pubic bone to the floor to stabilize your pelvis and to anchor your body to the floor. Before initiating movement, inhale slowly.

3. As you exhale, squeeze together your inner thighs and buttock muscles and bring your heels toward your buttocks.

DOUBLE LEG KICK
Figure 8.10

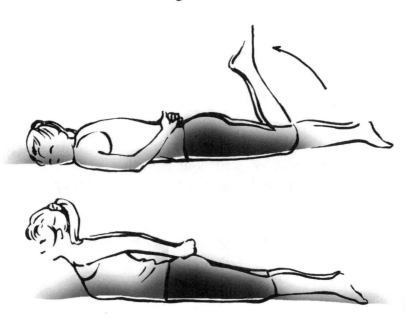

4. As you inhale, raise your chest off the floor and extend your hands (left hand still resting in right hand) behind you, palms facing the back of your head. At the same time, lower your legs to the floor. These two moves should be made in one fluid motion. Look at a spot on the floor a foot or so in front of you to keep your neck straight.

5. Exhale as you lower your chest to the floor, release your arms and return your hands to resting position on the small of your back. Rest the left side of your face on the floor. Repeat sequence five to ten times. Follow this exercise with Child's Pose on page 148.

Tips and Modifications

- To protect your back, keep your abs pulled to your spine, hips and pubic bone pressed firmly to the floor.
- Protect your neck—do not extend your head backwards when you raise your chest off the floor.
- If you feel pain in your knees, try decreasing the range of motion (i.e., don't bring your legs up so high).

- Feel the movement in your hamstrings, and visualize more length in your quads and hip flexors as you raise your legs.

Cautions: Don't do this exercise if you have back, shoulder, or knee problems.

Rating: II

SPINE TWIST

Benefits

Rotates the spine, stretches spine muscles, and facilitates exhaling breath to expel air fully before full inhalation.

Instructions

1. Sit on the floor with legs extended and together. Sit tall (on your sit bones) in good posture with abdominal muscles engaged, head held high, shoulders aligned over your hips, chest slightly raised, ankles flexed (extending through the heels).

2. Raise your arms so that they are extended from each side of the body and even with the shoulders, parallel to the floor. As you inhale, lift out of your hips, extending the spine and lifting tall, and exhale as you slowly rotate your torso to the left. Your hips should remain stable, and your

SPINE TWIST
Figure 8.11

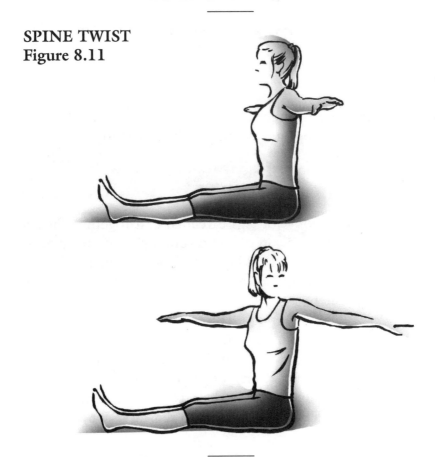

arms should remain extended from each side of your body. Visualize your rib cage rotating around your spine.

3. Return to the center with an inhaling breath, then as you exhale, rotate to the right, keeping abs engaged, arms even with your shoulders and parallel to the floor. Keep your chest open, and maintain good posture. Extend through the spine and keep neck relaxed and shoulders down from ears. Return to the center with an inhaling breath.

4. Repeat sequence five to ten times.

Tips and Modifications

• Most people will find it difficult to sit in this position. Sitting on a folded mat or blanket will lift your pelvis up a little bit so that you can sit without straining your legs. If you need to, you can place a small pillow underneath each knee for more support.

- You need to remain firmly connected to the floor from your sit bones to your heels throughout the exercise. Engaging your inner thighs will help you anchor your body to the floor during movement.
- As you move, you also need to feel extension through your legs. Keep your hips stable so that one leg doesn't extend farther than the other with movement. Visualize a plank of wood pressed against your abdomen. Your hips should remain in contact with the plank.

Caution: Move slowly to avoid strain.

Rating: II

SIDE KICK

Benefits

Increases strength and mobility in hip joints, works abdominal muscles, and stretches and strengthens thighs and buttocks.

Instructions

1. Lie on your left side with your head resting on your left arm, legs together. Bend slightly at the hips and move your feet forward one or two feet so that the body is slightly angled. Keep ankles slightly flexed. Place your right hand on the floor, palm down and fingers pointed in the same direction as your head, to form a "kickstand" that will help provide support for your trunk. Your kickstand should press up against your belly.

2. Pull your abs to your spine to stabilize your torso, and raise your right leg so that your feet are hips-width apart. As you inhale, use a slow, controlled motion to move your right leg forward, ankle flexed, keeping both legs straight.

SIDE KICK
Figure 8.12

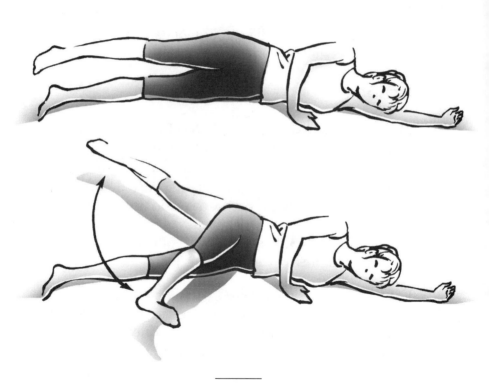

Keep your right leg (and inside edge of right foot) parallel to the floor throughout movement. Feel the stretch in the back of your right leg as you extend through your heel. You may feel a stretch in the buttocks (upper hamstrings), hamstrings, calves, and heel.

3. Still maintaining stability with your abs, exhale as you move your right leg backwards, behind the body, this time slightly pointing and reaching with your toes. Feel the extension in the front of your leg. You may feel a stretch through the front of hip, thigh, shin, and toes.

4. Repeat five to ten times. For a good side stretch, extend your raised leg back and reach up and in front of your face with your kickstand arm. Then repeat the exercise and stretch on the opposite side. Follow with Child's Pose on page 148.

Tips and Modifications

• Keep raised leg (and foot) parallel to floor throughout movement.

- Some people might find it more comfortable to lie in this position if they place a small pillow under the waist.
- Don't rely on your kickstand arm for support. You want to stabilize and hold your body in position using your core muscles.
- Your hips should remain stable, with top hip stacked above the bottom hip. Imagine that you have a steel rod that goes through both hips into the ground, and you can't move your hips forward or backward, or up and down. Imagine the same for your shoulders.
- To increase the challenge, when you move your leg forward, give it two pulses when you get to the end of your range of movement.
- There should be a small gap between your waist and the floor.

Caution: Be careful if you have lower back or hip problems.

Rating: II

SIDE LEG RAISES

Benefits

Strengthens obliques, thighs, hips, buttocks, and back muscles.

Instructions

1. Lie on your left side with your head resting on your left arm, and legs together. Legs can be slightly in front of the body, but not as angled as in Side Kick. Use right arm as support kickstand. Before initiating movement, inhale.

2. Exhale as you pull abs to spine to stabilize torso, and raise the right leg a bit past hips-width high, keeping it straight and toes slightly pointed. Extend through the toes. Keep hips stacked and stable.

3. Then raise left leg up until it presses against the right leg. Then slowly, as you inhale, lower both legs while maintaining balance and posture.

SIDE LEG RAISES
Figure 8.13

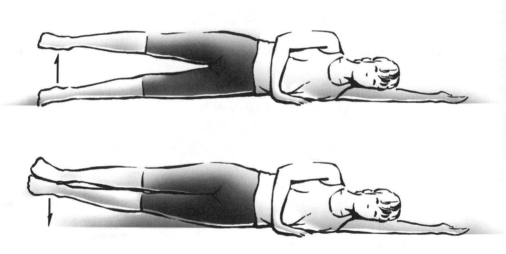

4. Repeat five to ten times, then repeat on the opposite side. Follow with Child's Pose on page 148.

Tips and Modifications

- Try this exercise with the body slightly bent at the waist, as in Step 1 of Side Kick.
- There should be a small gap between your waist and the floor. You can place a small pillow under the waist for support.
- Keep kickstand arm and shoulder relaxed.
- Maintain stability by continuing to pull abs to spine and engaging inner thighs.
- Don't forget to extend through the legs.
- Your head will remain resting on your arm throughout the exercise.

Caution: Be careful if you have lower back problems.

Rating: II

SWIMMING

Benefits

Provides cross-lateral training in the brain that facilitates right and left sides of brain working together, improving coordination. Strengthens and stretches spine muscles. Strengthens backs of legs, buttocks, and abs.

Instructions

1. Lie in a prone position, resting forehead on a small folded towel. (This position prevents you from straining your neck by keeping it in neutral position.) Place arms over head, palms down. Then rotate the forearms, still keeping them on the floor, so the thumbs are pointing to the sky. This movement shifts your shoulders into a more neutral position in which to perform the exercise.

SWIMMING
Figure 8.14

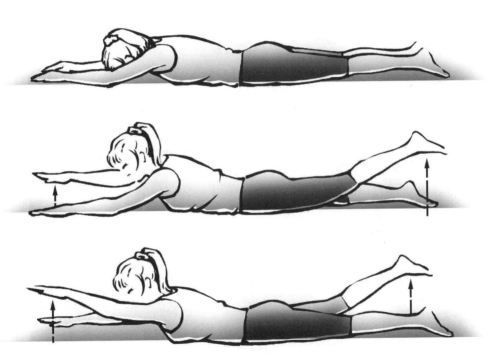

2. Pull your abs into your spine to stabilize your torso, and press your hips and pubic bone into the floor. Keeping your forehead on the towel, and your shoulders down and away from your ears, inhale as you raise your right arm and your left leg into the air, a few inches off the floor. Extend through your fingertips and toes.

3. As you exhale, lower your arm and leg and then raise your left arm and right leg, again extending through your fingertips and toes. Continue this sequence for five to ten times, inhaling for five counts and exhaling for five counts. Follow with Child's Pose on page 148.

Tips and Modifications

- To increase the challenge, raise your sternum off the floor as you raise your arm and leg. Look straight down to protect your neck.
- Keep your hips to the floor and your abs to your spine to support your lower back.

The Mat Exercises

- If the breathing instructions are too difficult, simply breathe normally throughout the movement.

Caution: Be careful if you have lower back problems.

Rating: II

CHILD'S POSE

Benefits

Relaxes and stretches the lower back; good to do after exercises that increase extension of the lower back.

Instructions

1. In a kneeling position, sit on heels.

2. Lower your chest to your thighs, then forehead to the floor, using your abs to control the movement and your arms to help support your weight. Let your arms stretch out in front of you, palms still touching the floor.

3. Bring your arms to your sides and rest them on the floor, hands toward feet, palms up. Rest in this position, breathing into your back. You will feel your ribs expand and the gentle stretch of the muscles around the ribs.

Rating: I

CHILD'S POSE
Figure 8.15

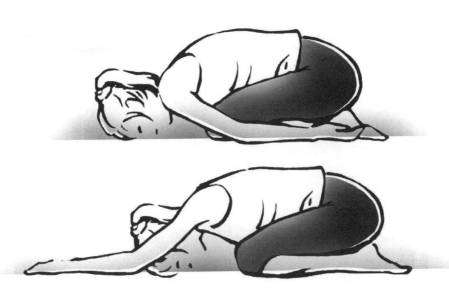

9 | Your Pilates Journey

Now that you understand the basics of Pilates exercises and philosophies, you're poised to begin your own Pilates journey. Hopefully, you've learned a new way of looking at exercise that makes you feel more in control of your body and your fitness routine.

Pilates is the perfect modern exercise. It's focused, effective, and efficient. Whether you're a busy person, a world traveler, or someone who doesn't want to join a gym or spend a lot of money on home exercise machines, Pilates provides a challenging workout that is adaptable to your individual needs.

As you progress with your Pilates routine, give yourself credit for being self-directed and disciplined enough to make a change in your life.

With time and practice, you'll become stronger, trimmer, and more flexible. And with your new physical strength comes more energy, confidence, and grace.

Add some Pilates to your life, and remember Joseph Pilates' motto, "Physical fitness is the first requisite of happiness."

Resources

For more information about Pilates, contact the businesses, organizations, and Web sites listed here:

Non-profit foundation for the Pilates community
The PilatesMethod Alliance
2631 Lincoln Ave.
Miami, FL 33133
Tel: 305-573-4946, 866-573-4945
www.pilatesmethodalliance.org

Education, teacher training and certification programs, Pilates classes, instructional videos, and Pilates machines and accessories:

Stott Pilates
2200 Yonge St., #1402
Toronto, Ontario M4S 2C6
Canada
Tel: 800-910-0001
www.stottpilates.com

The Pilates Institute of Australasia
PO Box 1046
North Sydney NSW 2059
Australia
Tel: 612-9267-8223
www.pilates.net

Education, teacher training and certification programs, Pilates classes, instructional videos, and teaching accessories:

PhysicalMind Institute
1807 Second St., Suite 40
Santa Fe, NM 87505
Tel: 505-988-1990
www.themethodfitness.com

Resources

Pilates machines, accessories, and instructional videos:

Balanced Body
7500 14th Ave., Suite 23
Sacramento, CA 95820
Tel: 800-240-3539
www.balancedbody.com

Peak Body Systems
5425 Airport Blvd., Suite 103
Boulder, CO 80301
Tel: 800-925-3674
www.peakbodysytems.com

Additional resources that provide information on Pilates, national and international instructor and studio directories, certification programs, class offerings, and equipment include the following Web sites:

- www.bodycontrol.co.uk
- www.mindbody.net
- www.pilates.co.uk

Index

INDEX

Index

INDEX

Index

INDEX

Index

INDEX

Index

INDEX